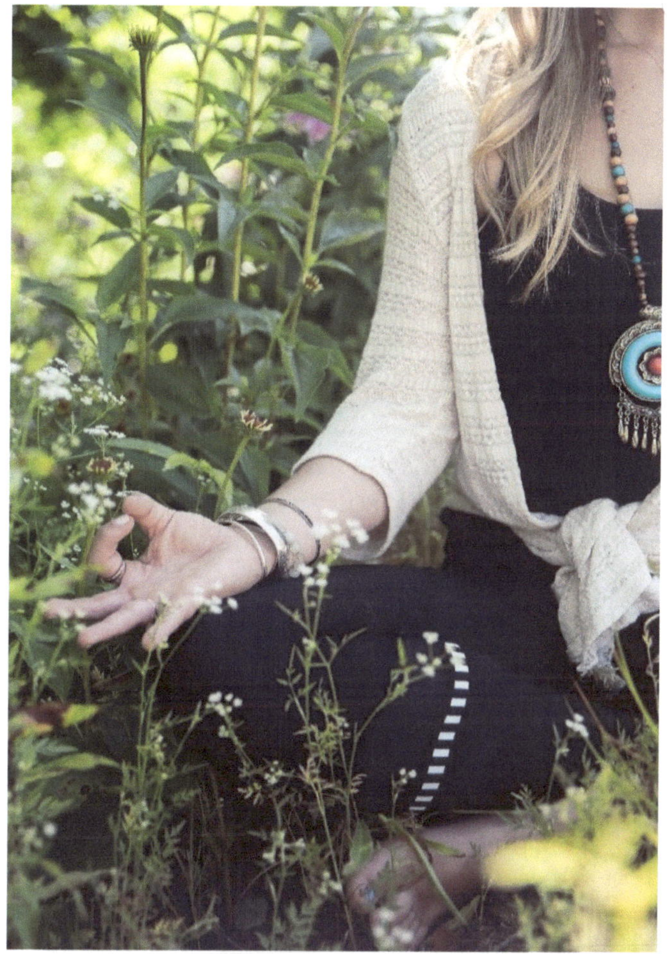

YOUR BODY IS IN LOVE WITH YOU

To me, "your body is in love with you" means your body will do anything you ask of it. If you ask it to sit in a chair all day, it will stretch, tighten and contort until your frame has been knotted into this perfect seated shape.

Yoga is here to help. With mindful breath, self-reflection, meditation, movement and all these other beautiful, helpful tools I have for you, we are able to reshape our bodies and our framework, promoting health and quality of life.

This book is filled with tips and tricks to keep you safe; specifically, during movement and breath, self-recovery and exploration time. The countless hours of sweating your heartaches out on your mat. The moments where you feel like you could expand east and west on your mat and onto the yogi's next to you...only then to remember your bum knee. This book is designed to teach you second nature cues and modifications to keep you safe in your body during your practice.

It is my hope that these teachings will keep you safe and returning to your practice for years to come.

DEDICATION

I dedicate this book first and foremost to my family. Thank you guys for my unconditional love, free legal consultations, editing, financial advice and full blown belief that it is 100% possible to follow and live out my dreams.

My UConn athletic training family that taught me most of this book and my Auburn sports medicine family that taught me how to apply it.

My EPIC tribe for guiding me through my first teacher training and all my Nashville loves.

Chel and Cec, my managers, social media advisors, all the love, laughs, singing at the top of our lungs and reminding me to let my hair down and laugh at myself!

Every single Soul to Sole patient, yoga studio and yoga teacher training, for believing in me and my power to educate and to heal.

To my love, Antonio…for without you, life would just be so much harder. For having dinner ready after my 13 hour works days, being my secretary when patients come early, grounding me when I've lost my mind…and so much more.

And lastly, to myself. YOU DID IT!!!

COPYRIGHT

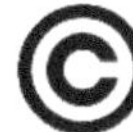 2018 Gabriella DeLorenze

Editors: Alexandra DeLorenze and
Julie "Beans" Burland

Proofreader: Anthony Cusimano

Photographer: Mary Craven Dawkins

Special editions or excerpts of Soul to Sole books can be created to specification. For details, contact Gabby at gabby@soultosolewellness.com

Find more of Gabby:
Website: www.soultosolewellness.com
Instagram: @soultosolewellness
Facebook: Soul to Sole Wellness

TABLE OF CONTENTS

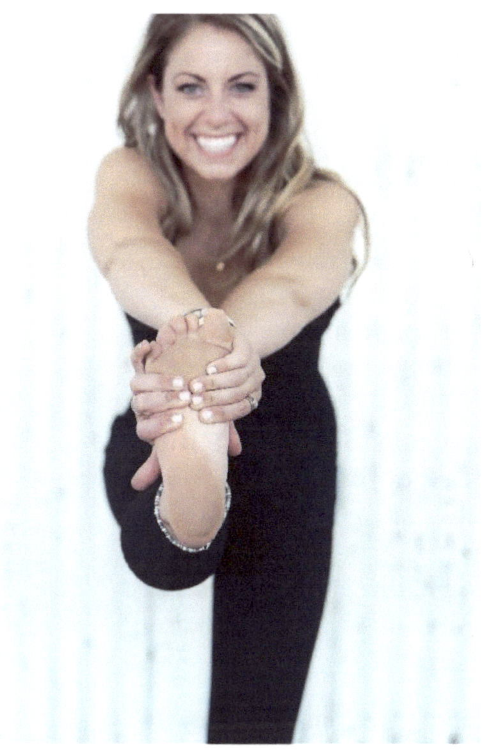

THE FOOT & ANKLE

People with flat feet will have more trouble keeping their knee tracking over their ankle (notice this by seeing the knee fall towards the center of the body with poses like crescent lunge*[10] /Warrior 2*[19]).

The CUEs:

"Ground down through your big toe and feel the arch of your foot lift"

"Press your knee toward your pinky toe"

"Engage the outside of your (R/L) hip and feel your knee open toward the outside of your body"

The most common pain in the feet that I see is in the plantar fascia. This "injury" or pain is referred to as plantar fasciitis: meaning, inflammation of the fascia or tissue on the bottom of your foot. Symptoms include stabbing pain near the heel. Pain may be worst in the morning.

To HELP:

Grab a tennis ball (or frozen water bottle!) and roll the bottom of your feet!

Sit in toes pose (in a kneeling position with your toes curled under) *[1] Remember to breathe! – Option to place a block between heels and booty to relieve some of the pressure.

Stretch your calves and hamstrings!! *[2]

Orthotics or a heel lift may help relieve pain throughout the day.

Strengthen your toes! Grab a towel. Using only your toes, curl and crunch until the towel is balled up at your feet. Spread out the towel, repeat! Have old marbles at your house? Pick those up with your toes too!

Your feet are your balance. Over 50% of your balance comes from your big toe alone! In every posture, bring attention to your feet first. Set the foundation before bringing your awareness up your body. Ground down through your big toes, feel the arches of your feet lift up and then feel the equanimity.

*[1] Please see Glossary for photo reference

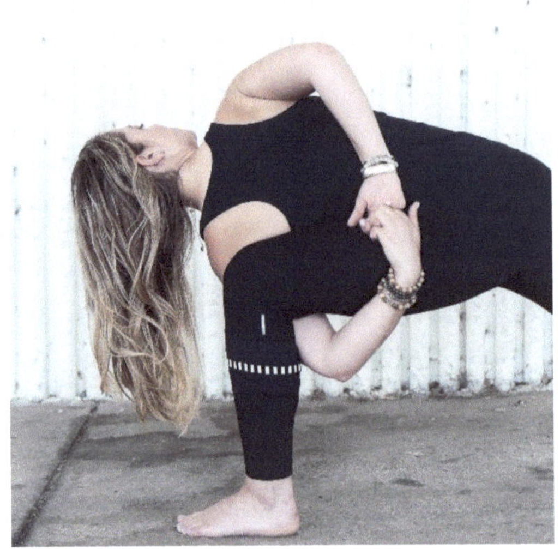

THE KNEE

Many people, including yogi's, have a hard time squatting. This is probably due to the way the majority of people sit day in and day out. However, this causes tight hips. These tight hips are the main reason for a lot of our knee pain.

To HELP:

Try a seated or reclined pigeon *3 on each side followed by a seated forward fold *4 and wide legged forward fold. *5

Stretch your hip flexors: low crescent lunge with arms up. *6

Open your quadriceps: lay on your side and reach back for your ankle (heel to booty) – for a bonus quadriceps stretch dorsiflex your foot (aka bring your toes closer to your shin). *7

TEACHERS TIP:

Remember the knee is a hinge joint! It's not built to sustain large rotational forces. Be careful when cueing students into big 180-degree movements to face the back of your mat.

The CUEs:
Example: Pyramid pose *8 from the front of your mat to the back of your mat:

"Ground through your heels and turn your toes to face the back of your mat"

"Keeping your quads engaged and knees straight, use your hips to bring yourself to face the back of your mat"

Be cautious to let the knees come over toes or falling into the middle of the mat in high and low lunge postures. Be aware in chair pose if the knees are coming over your toes; if they are, simply shift some weight back into your heels.

Engaging through your glutes (gluteus medius *9 specifically, but squeeze them all!) will help pull your knees out in squatting positions.

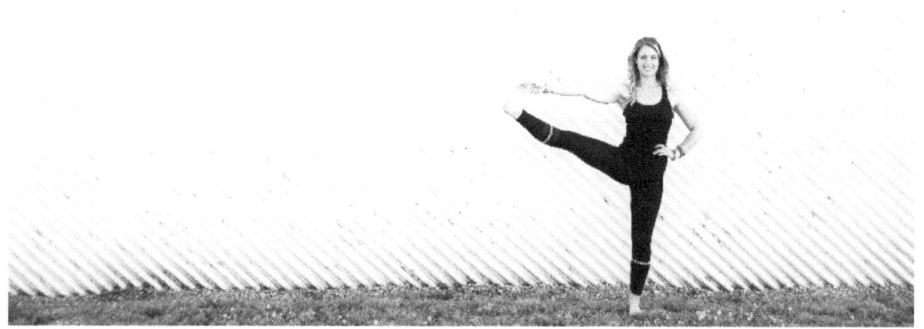

THE HIP

One of the #1 things that I love about yoga is that it makes you engage your glutes! A weak posterior line of your body (aka your entire backside) causes aches and pains and eventually, injuries.

Always remember to get your fair share of:
Crescent lunges *[10] – maybe add a few pulses up and down!
Bridge Pose *[11] – with holds and leg kicks and driving your knees forward as you squeeze your glutes!
Locust Pose *[12] – because strengthening your back as a unit is imperative.
>　　**Bring your big toes to touch (hip internal rotation) to help support a pain free locust

The hip is a ball and socket joint. It is meant to move about in all directions. With that being said, it never will "dislocate" without you knowing (aka excruciating pain). What you feel is probably your Iliotibial "IT" Band snapping over a spot on your femur (the greater trochanter for all my anatomy nerds out there!). Supine twist *[13], hug your knee into your opposite shoulder, release your glutes.

TEACHERS TIP:

Always remember the relationship the hip plays with the pelvis. Between the hip flexors, the hamstrings, the latissimus dorsi and the glutes there's a lot of pushing and pulling going on. Everyone will be a little different but play with toes in/toes out *aka: hip internal and external rotation*.

The CUEs: Example poses:
Airplane *[14]**/Standing splits** *[15]**:**
"Let your back toes face the ground"
"Square your hips to the floor"

Downward facing dog *[16]**:**
"Bring your toes in, heels out (& in!)"

Wide legged forward fold *[5]**:**
"Bring your toes in/heels out"

"Play with rocking the weight into your toes, feel the difference in your hamstrings"

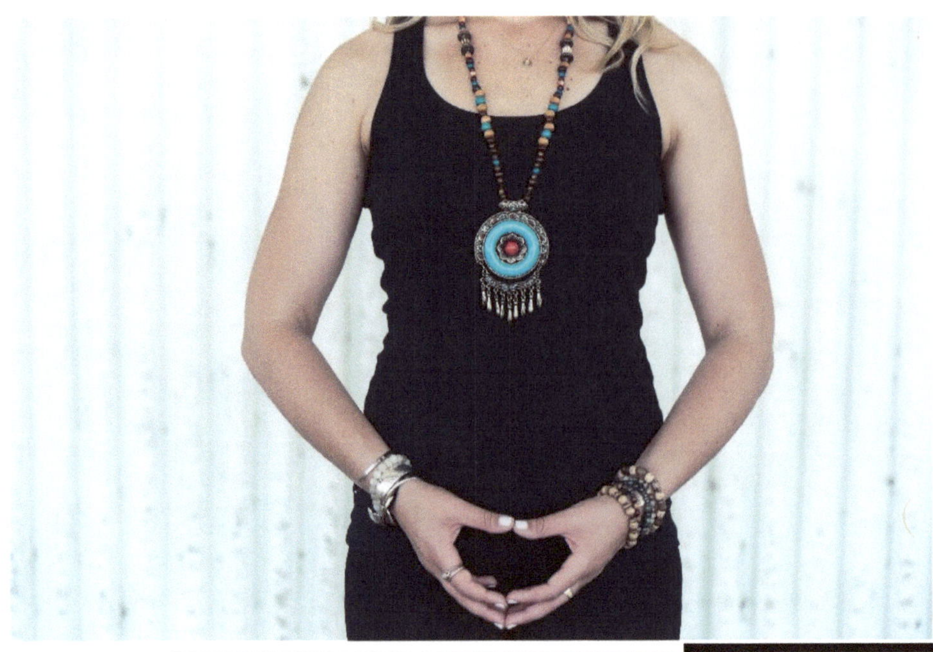

THE PELVIS

The pelvis is your center of gravity/center of mass. It holds so many vital organs and therefore, a lot of energy. Tightness, weakness and imbalances are no stranger to the pelvis.

The diagram to the left shows what I most commonly see in yogi's: tight hip flexors, tight low back with weak abdominals and glutes. This commonly leads to an increase in their kyphotic (mid-back) curve and a forward head posture.

To HELP:

With all core exercises, get great at holding a posterior pelvic tilt.

"Tuck your pelvis under" or "bring your low back to the mat"

Supine Heel Taps *21:
Lay on your back, stack knees over hips, feet flexed towards your face. Bring your arms up to the sky and flatten your lower back into the ground. Mula Bandha! From here, hinging at the hip, try dropping one heel to the ground. Bring it back to meet the other leg, switch sides, repeat.

TEACHERS TIP:

Posterior pelvic tilt will protect the low back in during back extension postures but know that anterior pelvic tilt will help you open more.

The CUEs:
Bridge pose *11 prep:
"Press your low back into the ground"

Chair pose *17:
Avoid increase anterior pelvic tilt (see this as big low back arch)
"Pull your belly button into your spine"
"Tuck your pelvis under"
"Slightly flatten your low back"

Warrior 1&2 *18/Crescent *10/all split stance asana:
Avoid low back arching, especially with shoulders flexed overhead.
"Pull your front hip back and press your back hip forward"
+ CHAIR POSE CUES

Imagine your hips are a jug of water. If the water falls out the front, it's anterior pelvic tilt. *19 If the water falls out the back, it's posterior pelvic tilt. *20

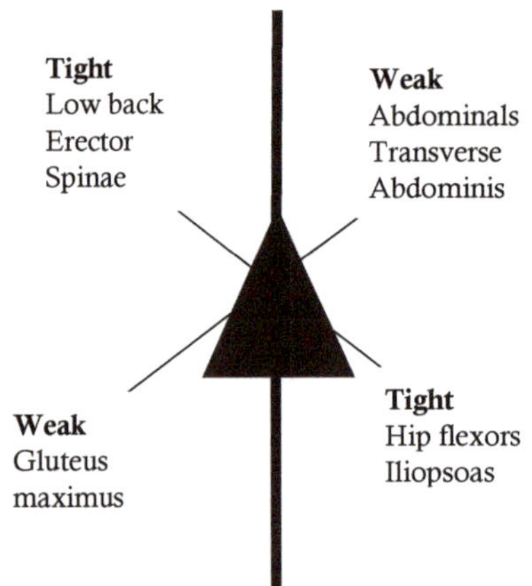

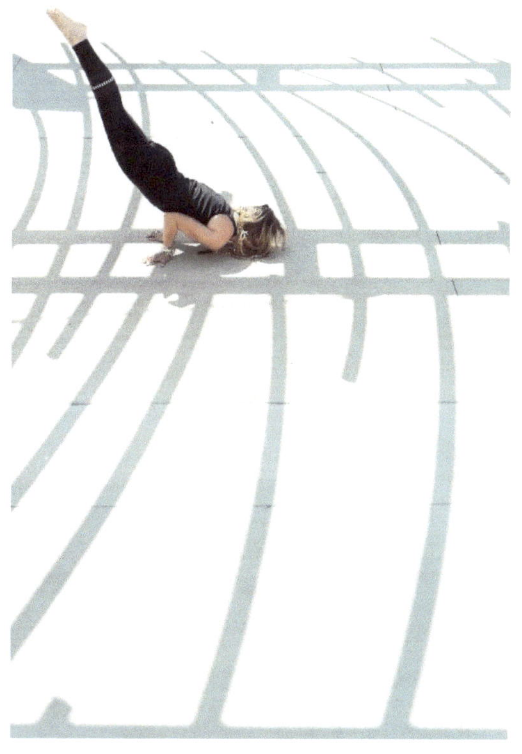

THE SPINE

Low back pain is BY FAR one of the #1 reason why yogi's seek my help. Low back pain is the #1 reason why 80% of Americans seek orthopedic MD's as well.

To HELP:
Practice a "dead bug" position *22:

- On back
- Knees bent stacked over hips, feet up and flexed towards face
- Arms to sky
- Flatten lower back to ground
- Pull belly button to spine
- You can hold here (30sec- 1 min), add in a crunch to the sky, lower one heel to the ground (be sure to hinge at your hip keeping knee bent) and then repeat

The main goal is that you keep your low back on the ground throughout the entire sequence on your back! Belly button pulled into your spine, mula bandha engaged, transverse abdominis turned on!

Remember breakfast, lunch and dinner to remember how many vertebrae you have:

Breakfast (7am): Cervical spine = 7

Lunch (12pm): Thoracic spine = 12

Dinner (5pm): Lumbar spine = 5

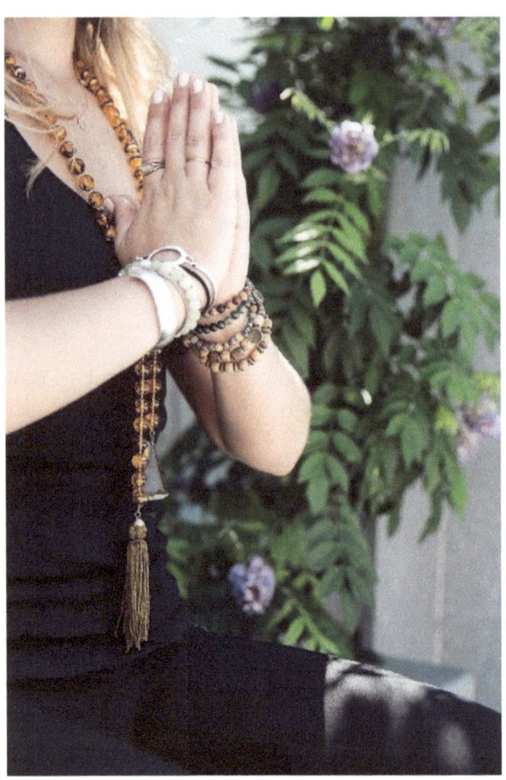

THE DIAPHRAGM

The diaphragm is a dome shaped muscle that lines the insides your ribs and almost looks like a sideways "C" as the middle of the muscle sits up into your rib cage. As you INHALE it contracts and shortens as you EXHALE it relaxes and goes back to its dome shape to help press the air out of your lungs.

The reason you get the hiccups is because your diaphragm is "out of whack" from your breath.

TEACHERS TIP:

Be sure to cue the breath. Especially as the flow gets harder and your students become more fatigued.

The main goal with cuing the breath is to guide your students deeper into a moving meditation and out of the sympathetic nervous system.

To Keep in Mind:

Belly breath works WAY BETTER than chest breath!

There should be ZERO upper trapezius (top of your shoulder by your neck) movement when you breathe.

You should be able to keep the core in tight, ribs knit together and still breathe normally.

To build heat, breathe in and out through your nose (ujjayi breath) it's loud, powerful, ocean wave sounding.

To release heat, open your mouth and lion's breath or a simply loud "sigh" or exhale out your mouth.

Remember: Your heart rate is involuntary. The best way we can control the heart rate is to control the breath!

Be cautious if any of your students are on a beta blocker – you will want to keep the heart rate low! (Make sure any student you have that is on a beta blocker has a heart rate monitor on!).

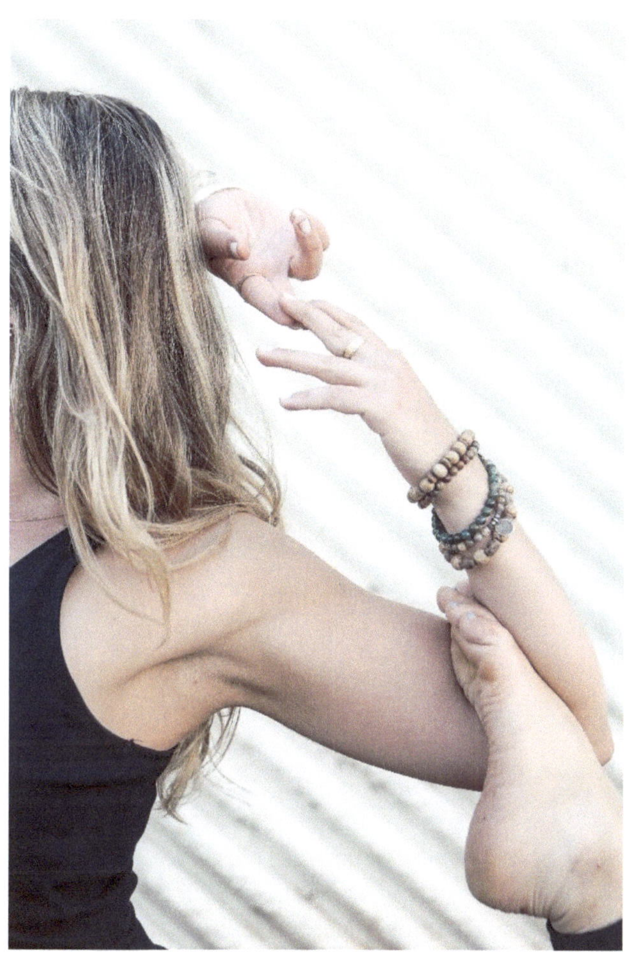

THE SHOULDER

For your practice, it is imperative to find strength and stability in the shoulders. In chaturanga, always remember to never dip the shoulders below the elbows. Pain in Warrior 2? Try bringing the palms up to the sky. Always remember: Yoga, especially vinyasa, works a lot of "push" muscles. Remember to work the "pull" muscles as well. Work on lowering slowly into chaturanga *25 and then pressing back up!

The biggest shoulder aches and pains that I see in my clients are due to:

#1: Lack of internal shoulder rotation *26

To HELP: While holding a strap, reach hand around to your low back. Take the strap over the opposite shoulder and pull up to feel the stretch.

#2: Poor posture

To HELP: Strength your back muscles. Exercises that help: Cable rows *27, bent over rows *28, Lat pull down machine *29.

THE ELBOW

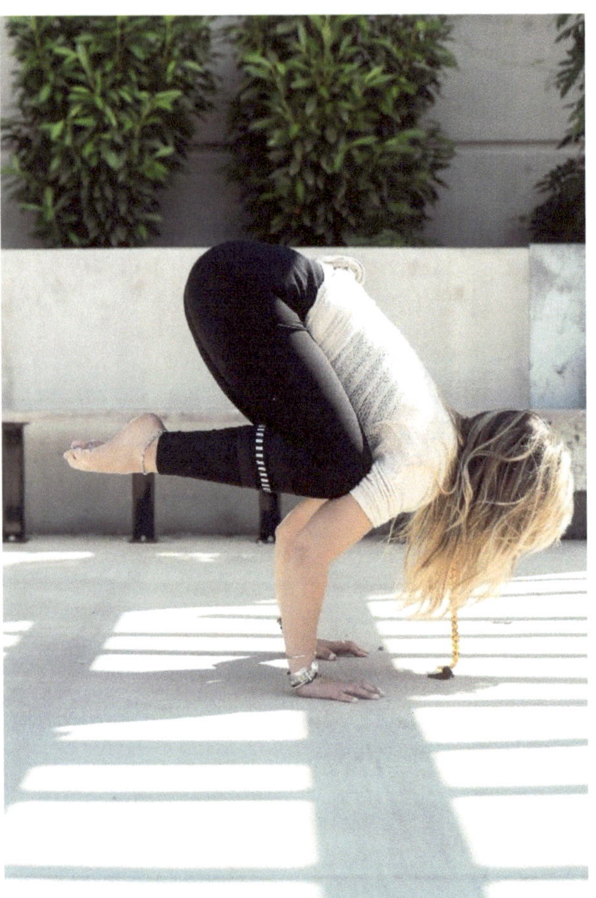

Most common pain I see in the elbow is tendinopathy (-opathy = denotes a disease or disorder) on the inside (medial) or outside (lateral).

To HELP:

1. Increase your shoulder mobility and your scapular control. Just as the hips control your knee, the shoulder 100% effects the pulls and movement of your elbow and wrist. Posture plays a huge role here too!
2. Check wrist mobility one side compared to the other side.
3. Friction massage: the wrist flexors (bringing your fingers toward the inside of your forearm) insert on the medial (inside) elbow, the wrist extensors (bringing your fingers away from the inside forearm) insert on the lateral (outside) elbow. Take 2 fingers. Find a spot that's tender and for 4 minutes vigorously rub side to side. Ice after if sore. A fun way to ice: Freeze a paper cup filled half-way with water. Rip off the top of the cup to expose the ice and continuously rub over the entire effected area!
4. Spend less time on the computer/balancing on your hands/driving. Limiting your favorite movements and postures help significantly. decrease all tendinitis as it is an overuse injury.

TEACHERS TIP:

Your flexible students may hyperextend at their elbows. This is noticeable with a posture like crescent lunge *10 with arms extended overhead and most especially in downward facing dog. *16 Now here's the muddy part: some anatomists don't mind this as it is their proper range of motion. Here's my thoughts: if you're not in "alignment" aka hyperextending, there is probably a bone-on-bone situation going on at your joint. Over time, this will lead to aches and pains and further hyperextension!

The CUEs:

"Bring space to your elbow joint"

"Soften the inside of your elbow"

"Feel your bicep engage as you press away from the mat"

Your elbow is a hinge joint (like the knee) with a slight rotation (supination or palms up and pronation or palms down). Notice in a pose like downward facing dog *16 if your elbows face the front of the room. Notice how you can bring the inside your elbows to face each other. Then notice how this motion is PROBABLY coming from your shoulder!

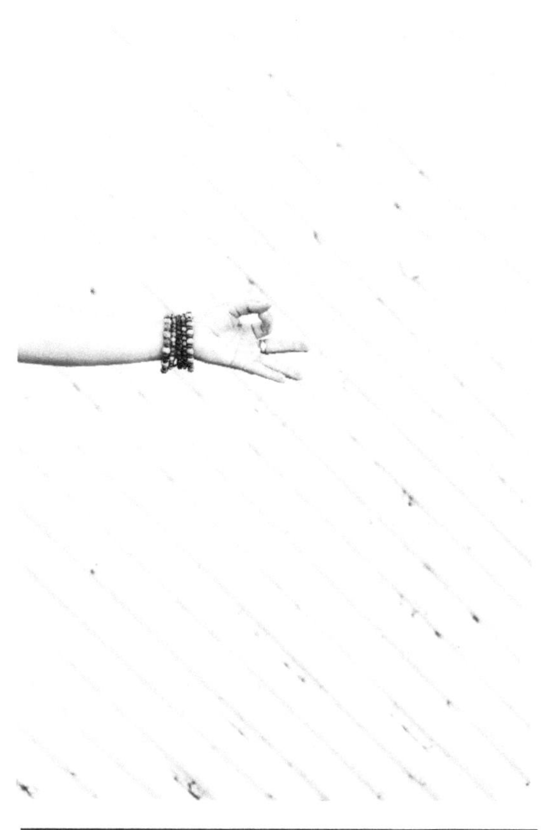

THE HAND
& WRIST

Always remember to have live and active fingers in all of your postures. This will help strengthen the wrists and elbow.

Place your thumb and index or middle finger around your wrist. Notice the space between the tips of your fingers. Make a strong close fist. Notice the space change. Make your fingers wide. Again, notice the changes. Make your fingers long but touching. To strengthen your wrists, you want to feel your muscles engaged. Every yoga posture is an opportunity to strengthen your wrists.

Try and limit closed fists. We are energy: a closed fist is a closed circuit.

The biggest pains I see in yogi's in the hands and wrists are indebted to inversions. Due to increased time spent on your hands with your wrists bent (extension).

To HELP: Find a stress ball, putty or a big bucket of rice and squeeze and relax and squeeze and hold and relax…this strengthens the surrounding wrist muscles.

To HELP: Your wrist extensors and flexors insert at your elbow. Try rubbing on the inside and outside of your elbow to help release your wrists.

To HELP: Work on having good supination and pronation. This is when you bring your palms to the sky and palms down. Rest your forearm off the edge of a table and hold one end of a dumbbell. Let the dumbbell fall to one side brining your palm to the sky. Hold for the stretch. Bring back through center and fall palm down. Hold and repeat.

Based off this information you have a lot of great cues and things to keep in mind while you're teaching and taking future yoga classes.

And great cues lead to stronger muscles.

And stronger muscles lead to less injuries.

And less injuries lead to more yoga.

And more yoga leads to more peace.

(& for teachers: less injuries = more students = more money!)

When you are physically practicing yoga, the last thing you want on your mind are aches and pains…allow my book to help guide you through a journey closer to your authentic PAIN FREE self.

With simple anatomy, you can keep yourself and your students safe.

Please let me know what you need and how I can be of service.

Namaste and all my Love,

Gabby

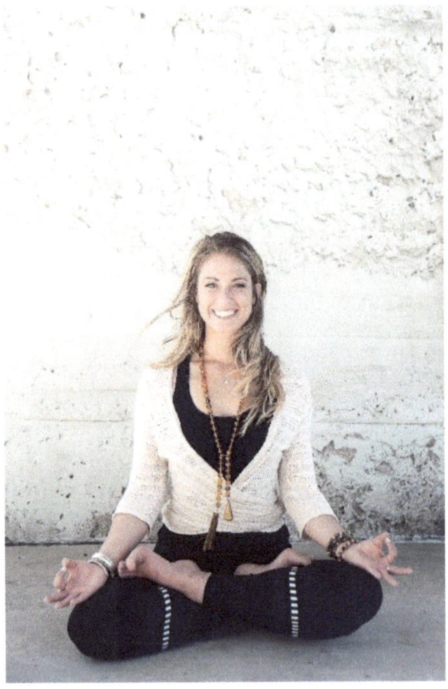

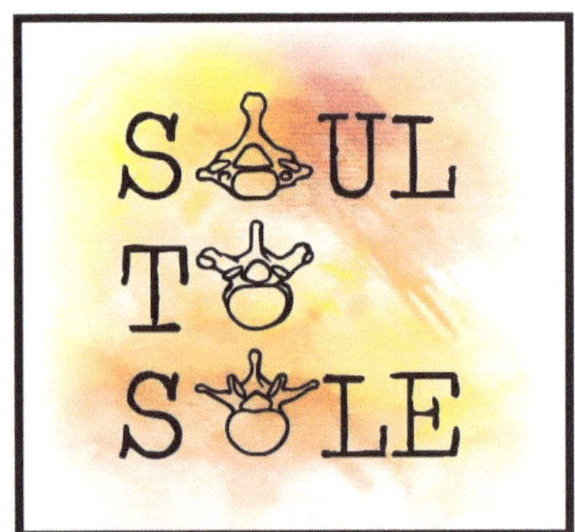

www.learnyogaanatomy.com

GLOSSARY

1.   Toes Pose

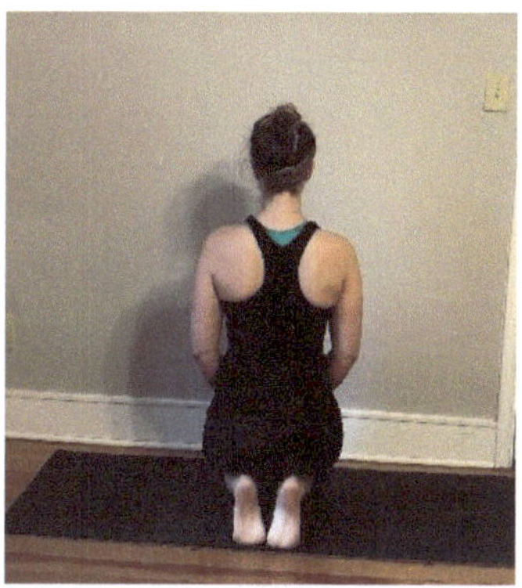 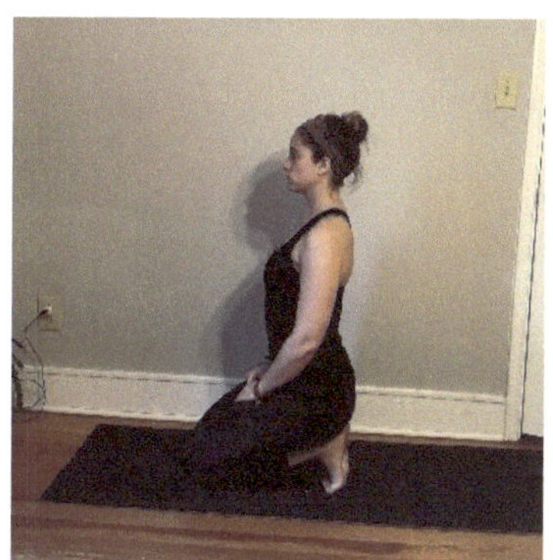

2.   Calf/Hamstring Stretch

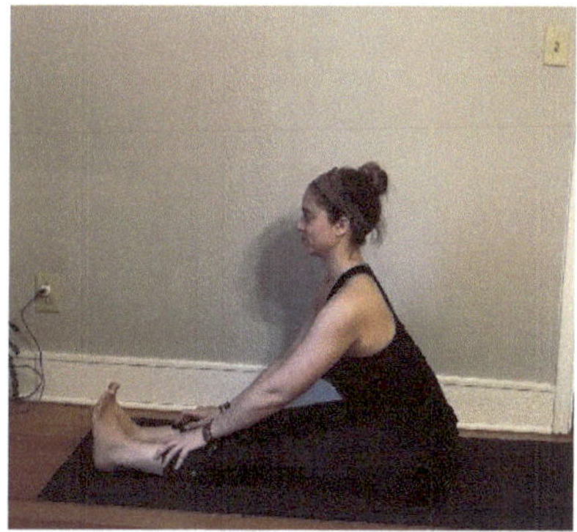 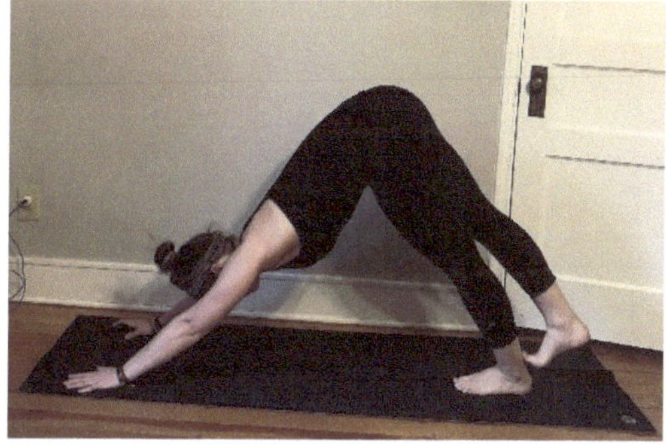

3.   Reclined Pigeon

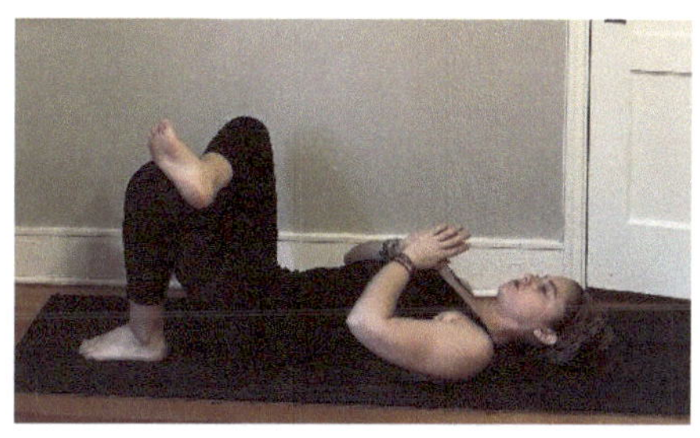 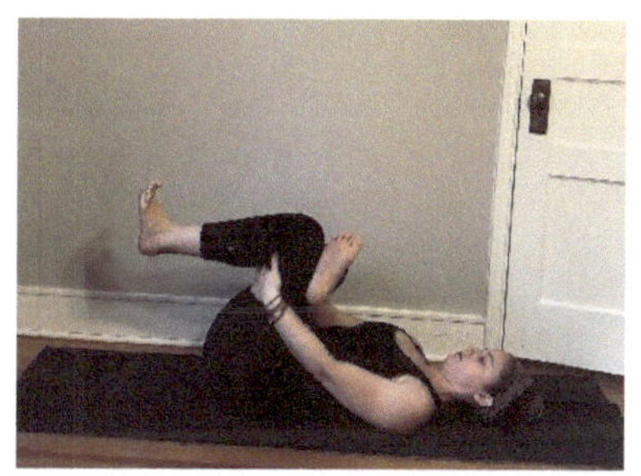 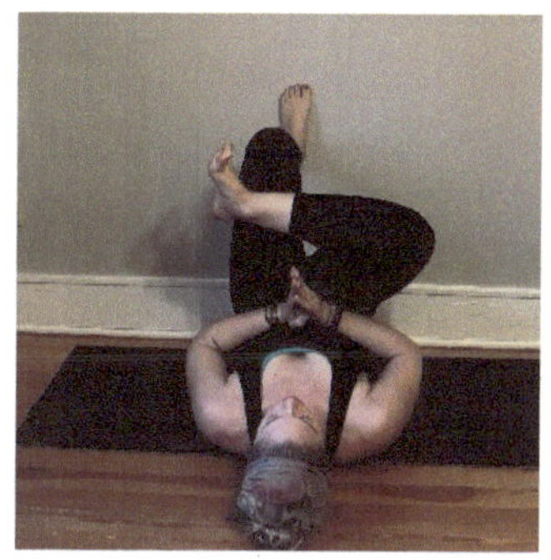

4.   Seated Forward Fold

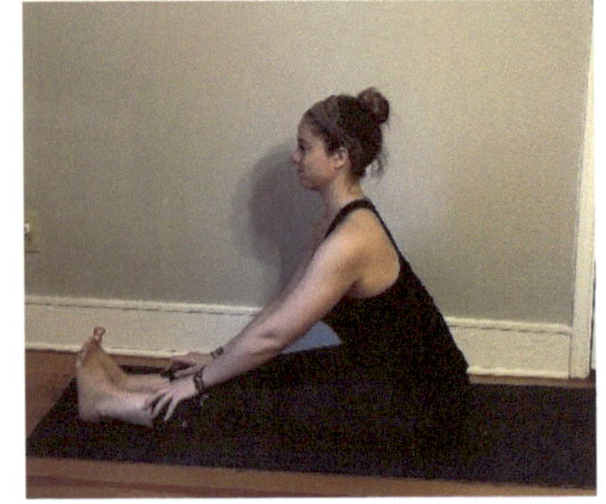 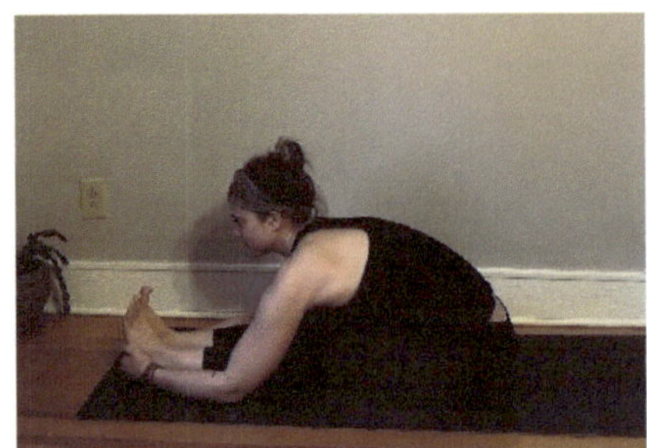 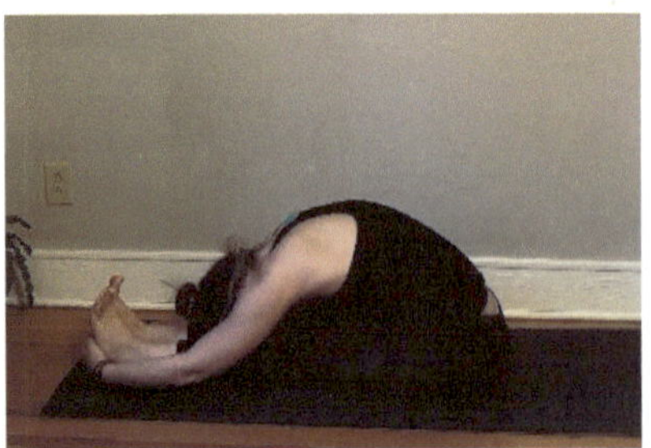

---

5.   Wide Leg Forward Fold

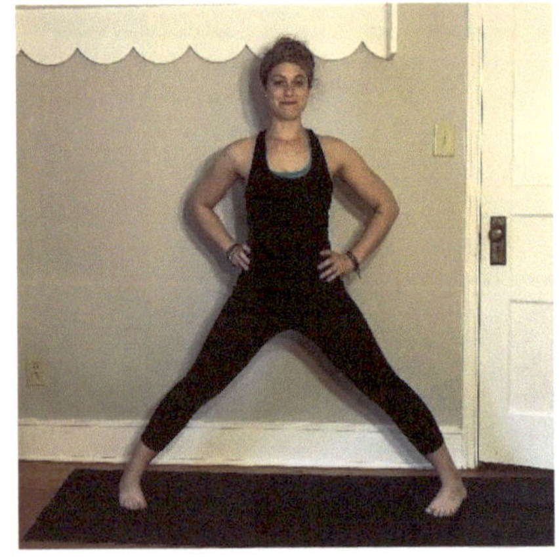 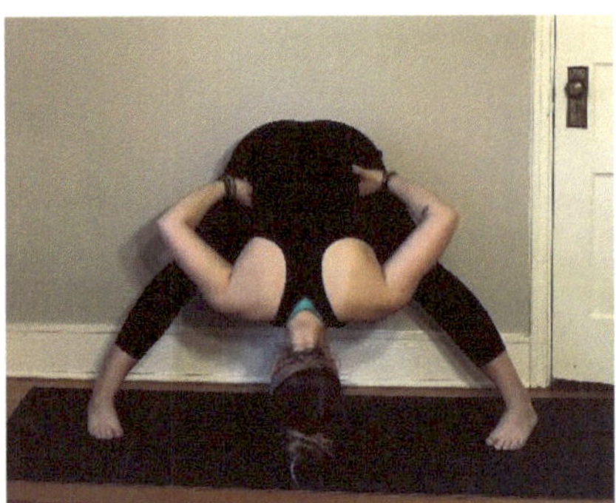 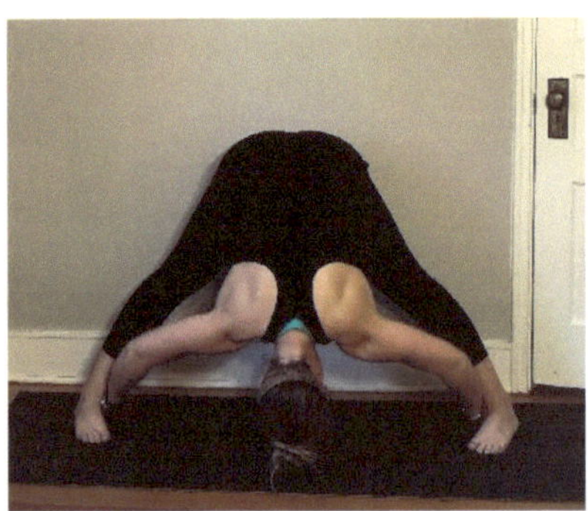

---

6.   Low Crescent Lunge

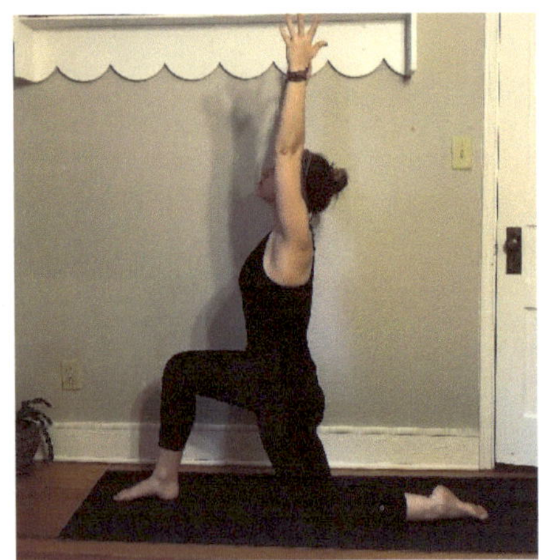

7.   Quadriceps Stretch

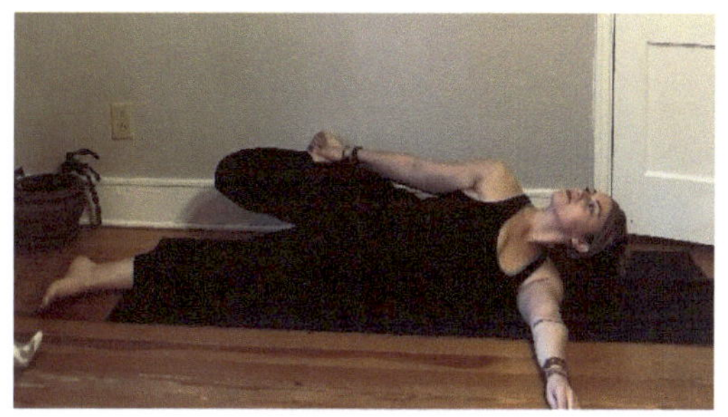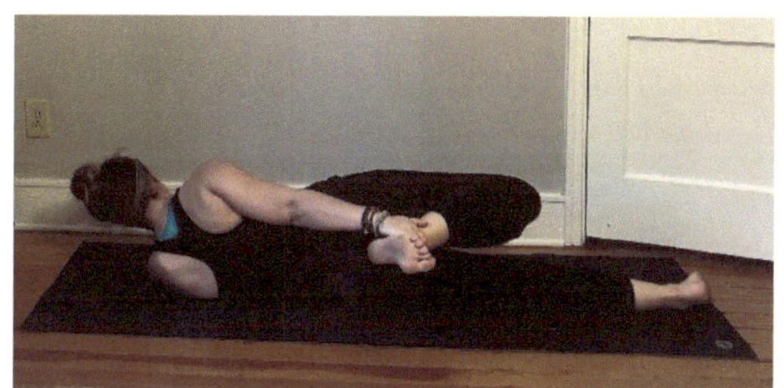

8.   Pyramid Pose

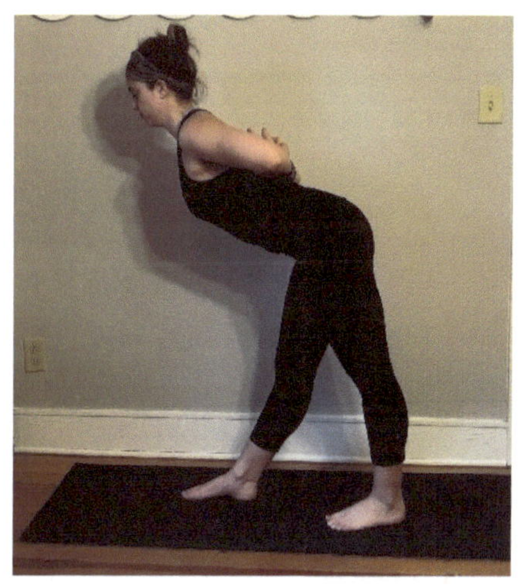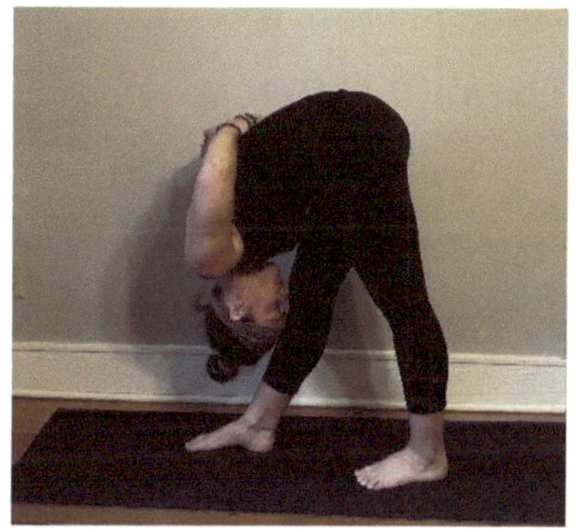

9.   Gluteus Medius Muscle

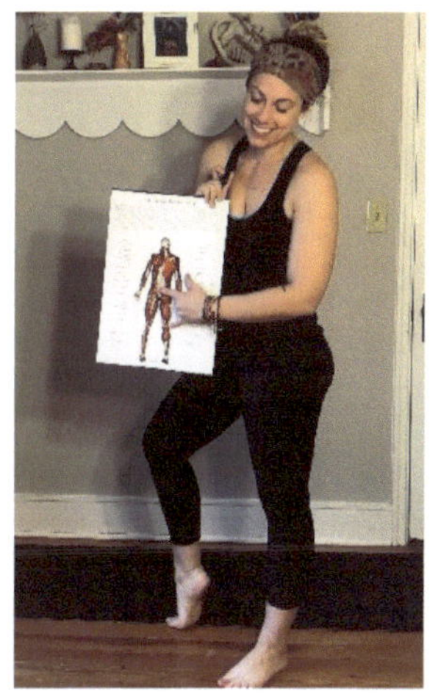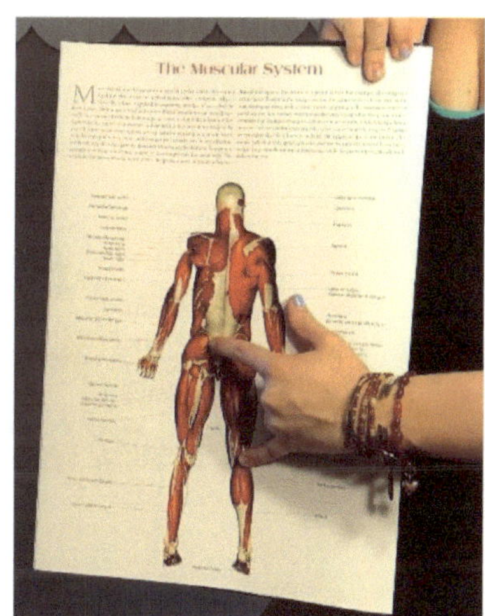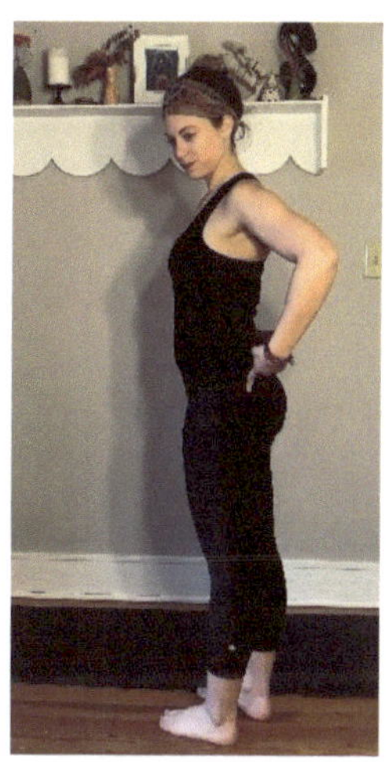

10.   Crescent Lunge (into the split squats)

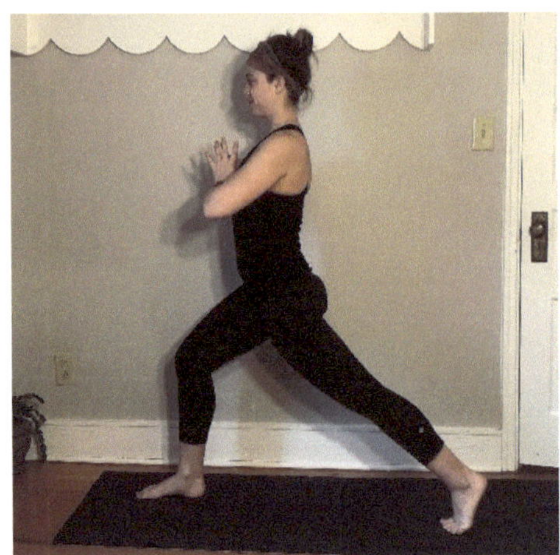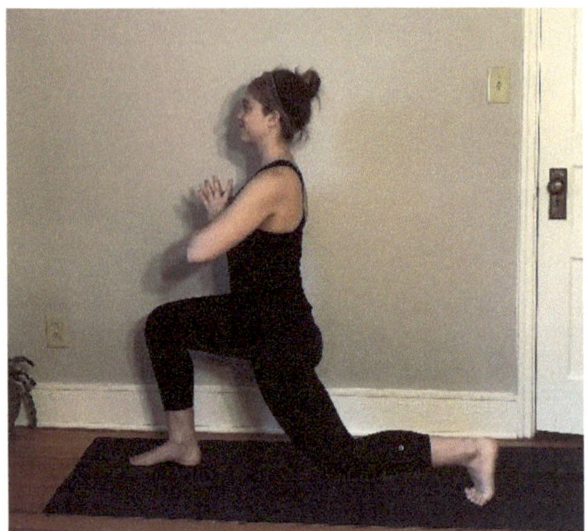

---

11.   Bridge Pose

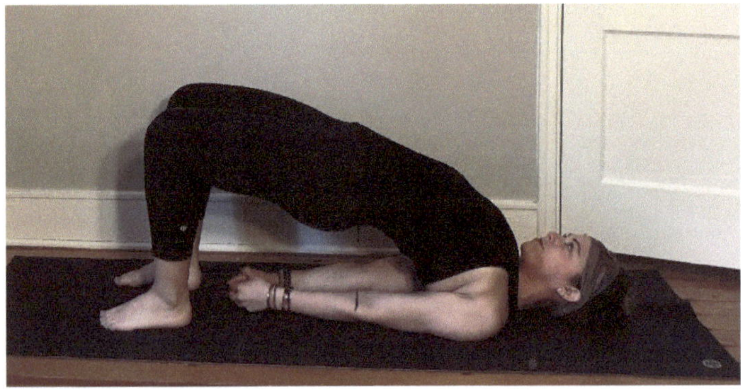

---

12.   Locust Pose

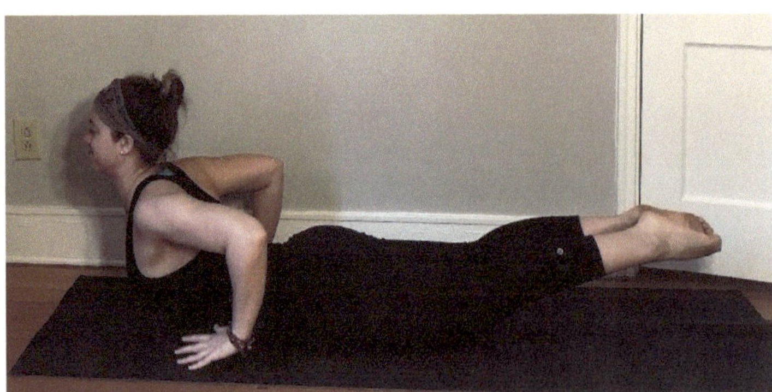

13.   Supine Twist

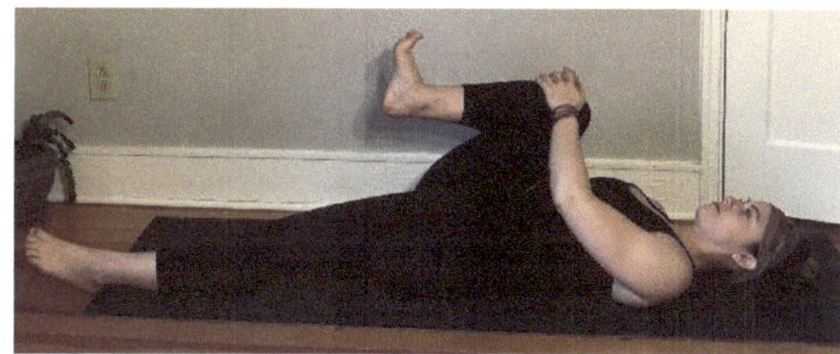 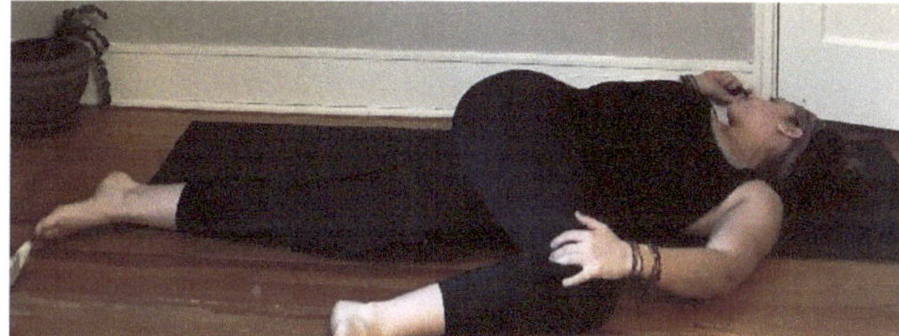

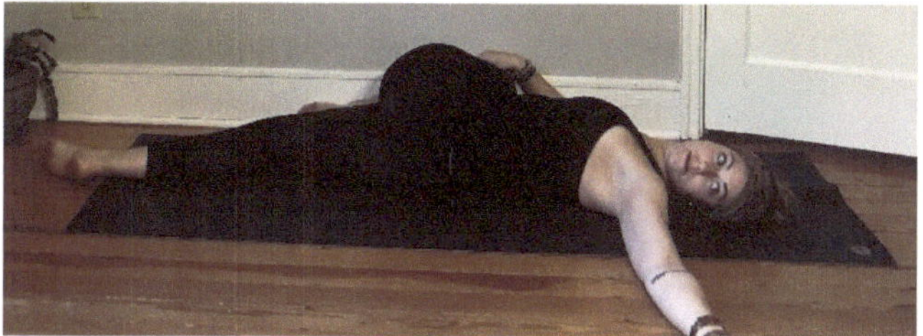

14.   Airplane

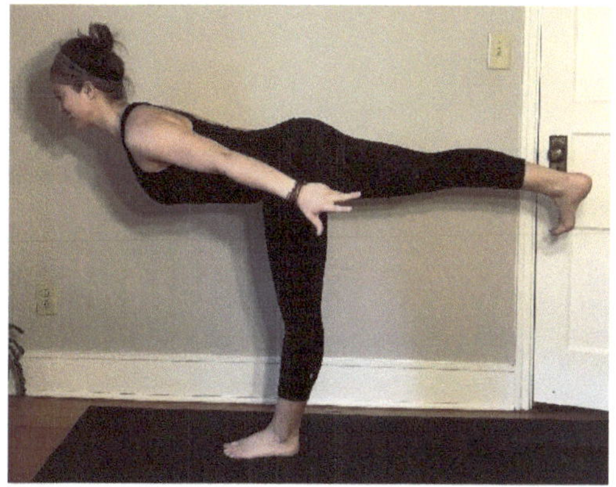

15.   Standing Splits

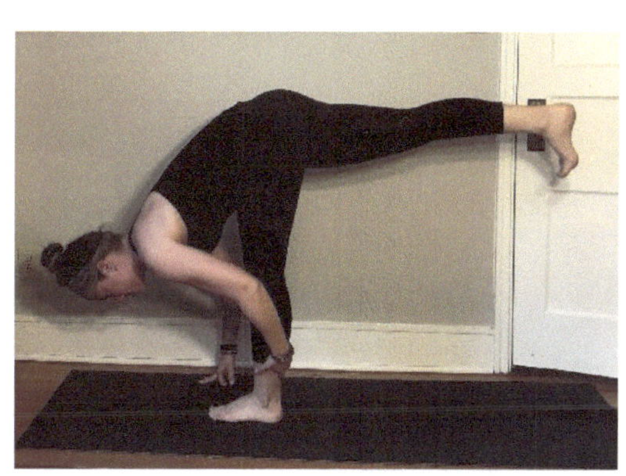 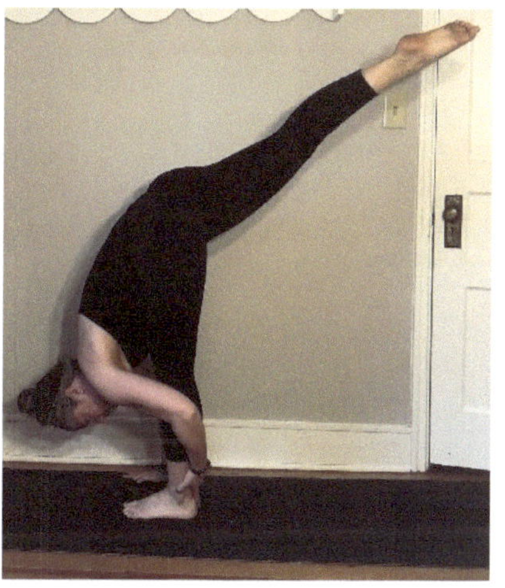 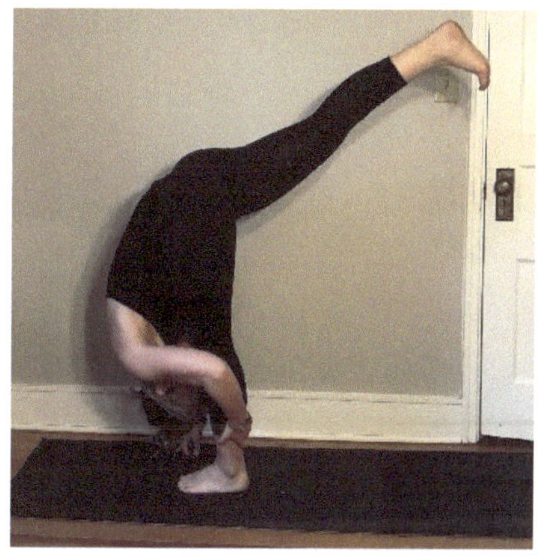

16. Downward Facing Dog

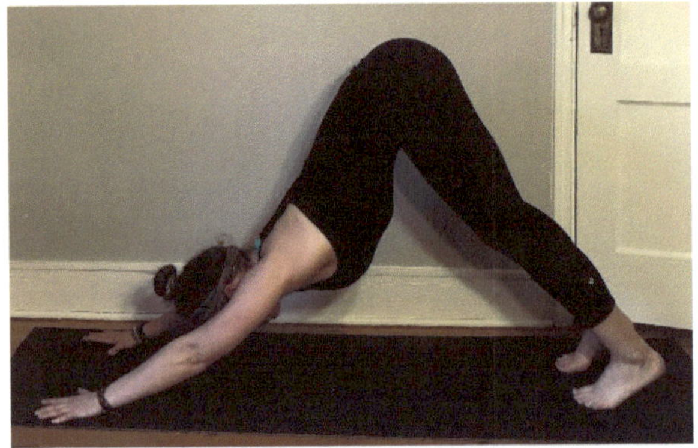

---

17. Chair Pose

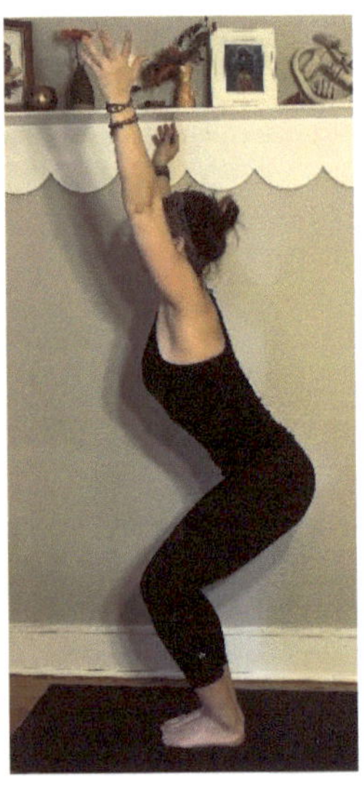 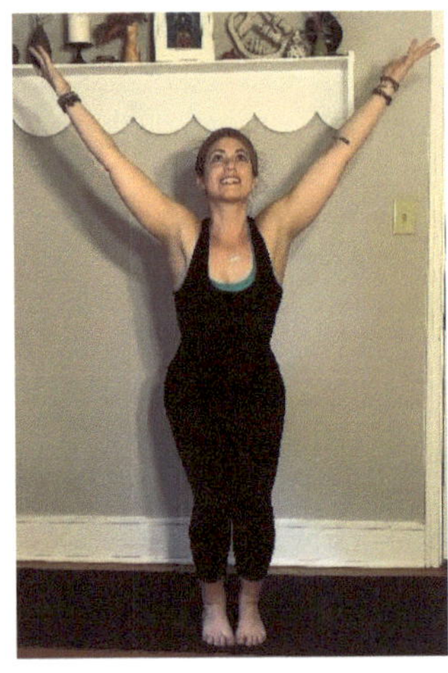

---

18. Warrior 1 & Warrior 2

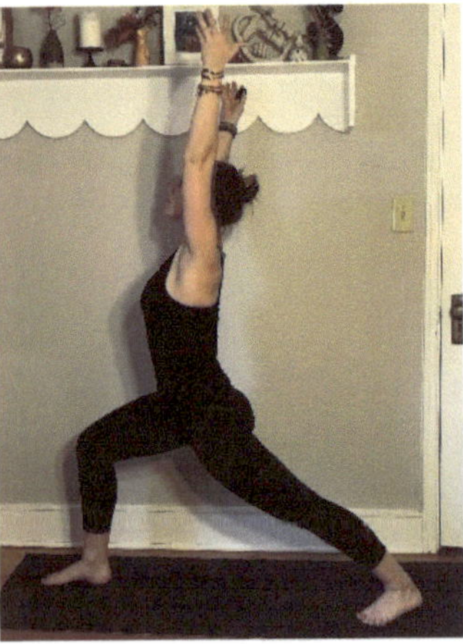 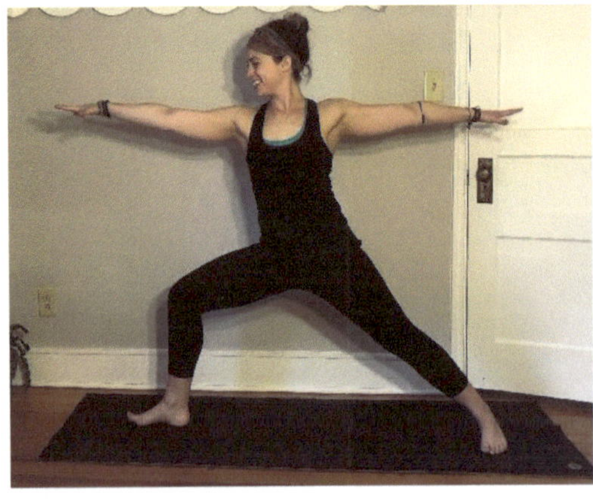

19.   Anterior Pelvic Tilt   **20.   Posterior Pelvic Tilt**

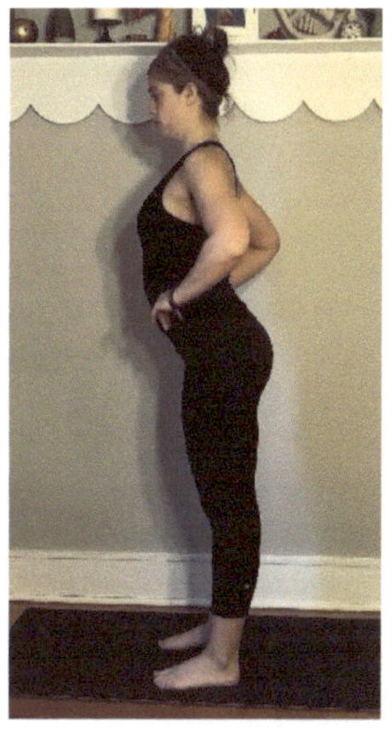
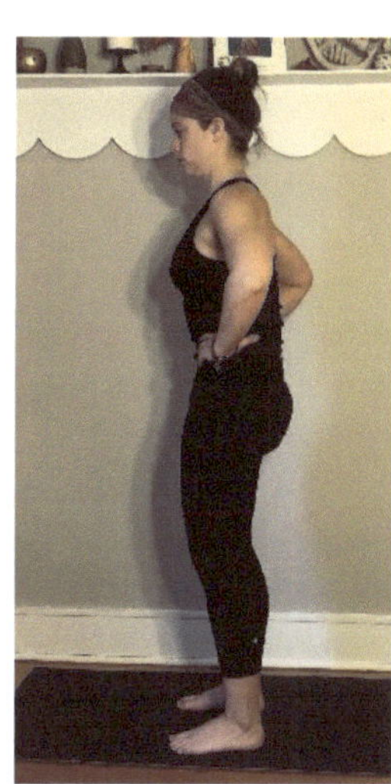

---

21.   Supine Heel Taps

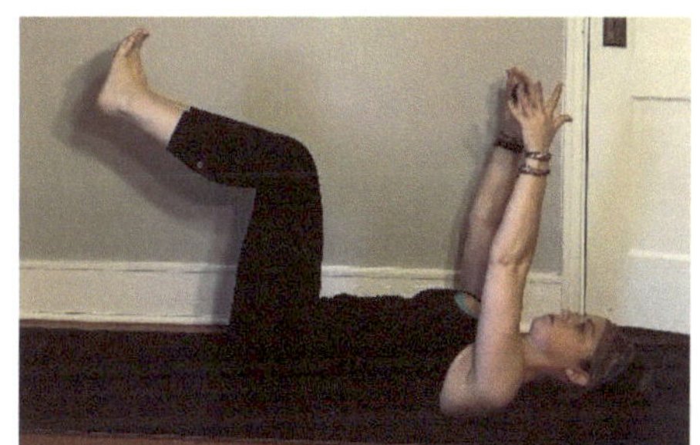
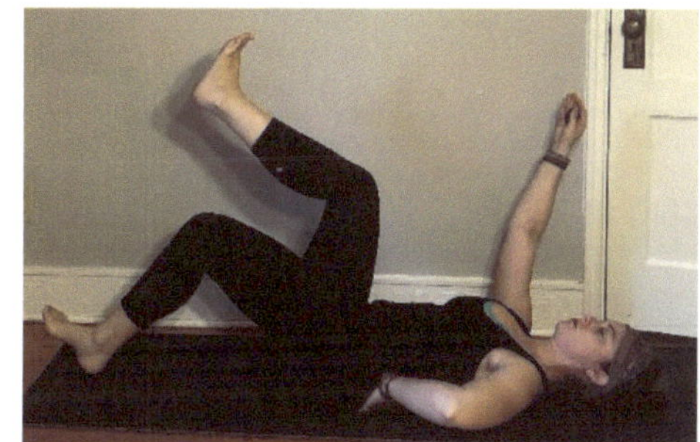

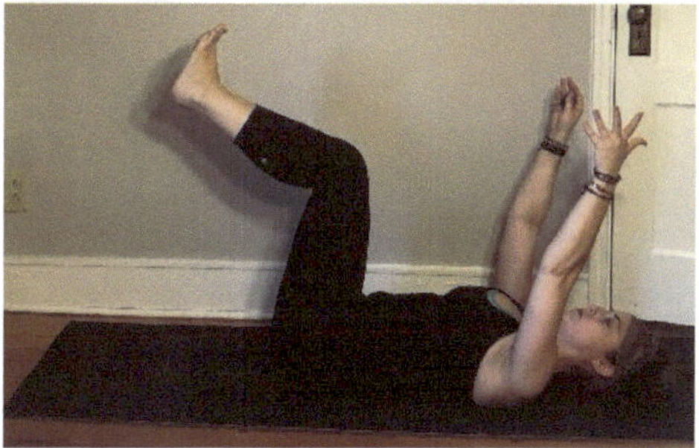
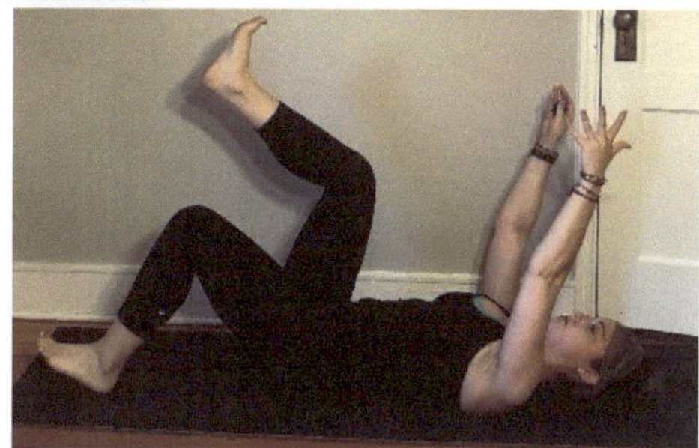

---

22.   DeadBug

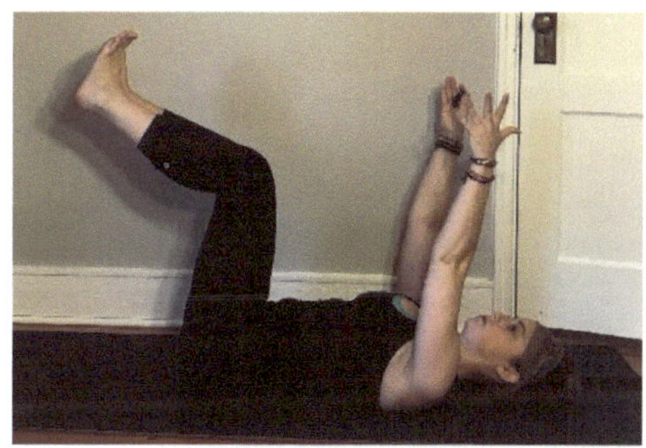

---

23. **Wheel Pose**

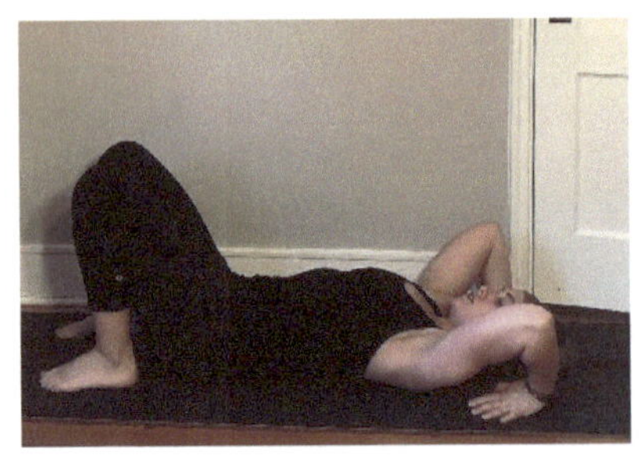 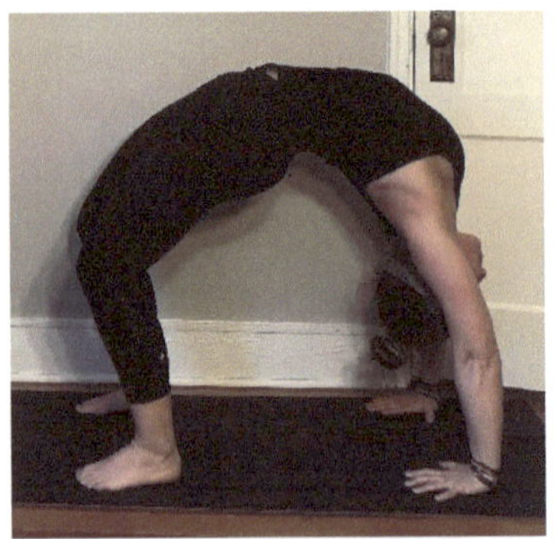 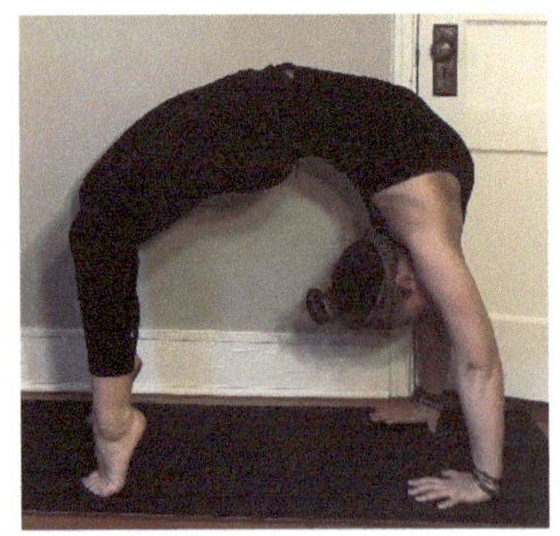

24. **Floor Bow**

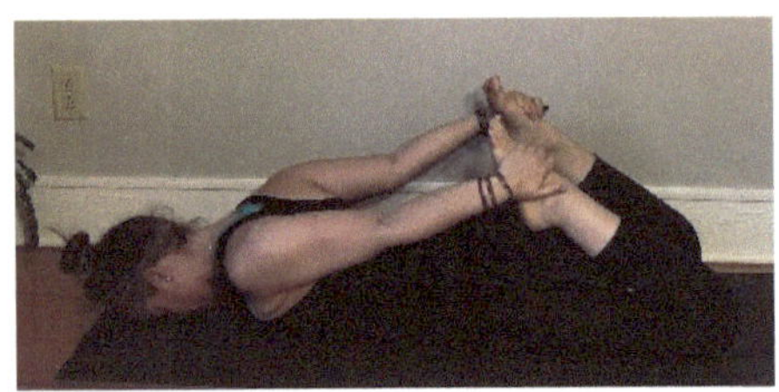 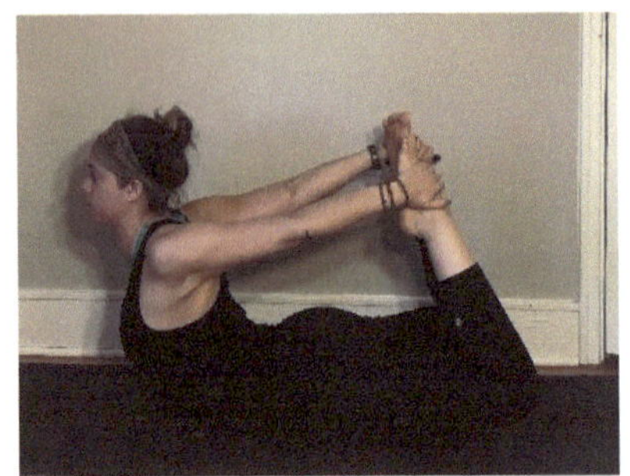

25. **Chaturanga**

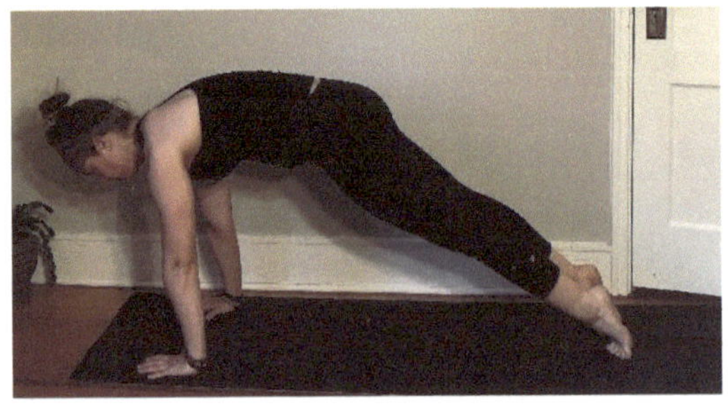 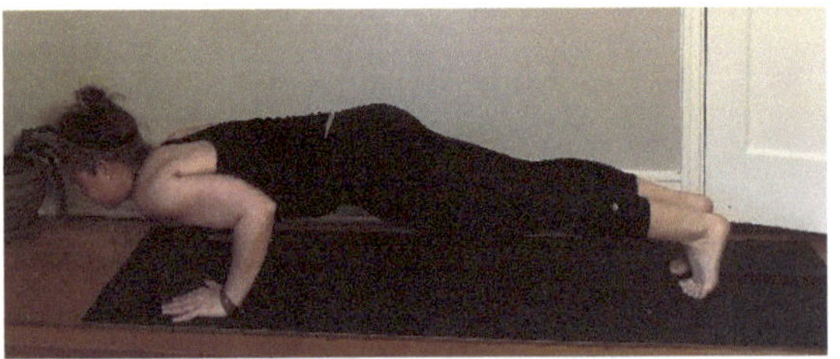

26. **Internal Shoulder Rotation**

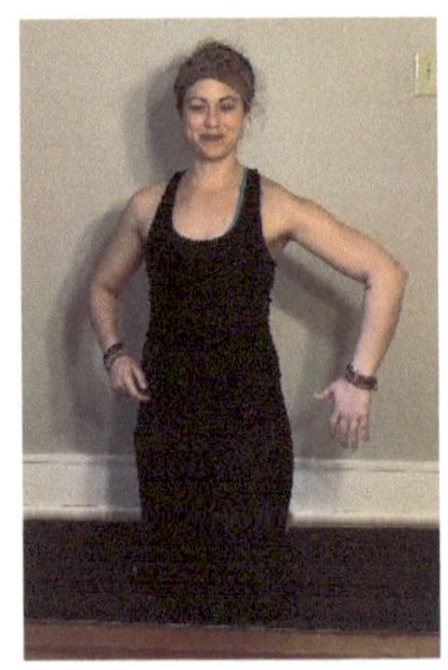 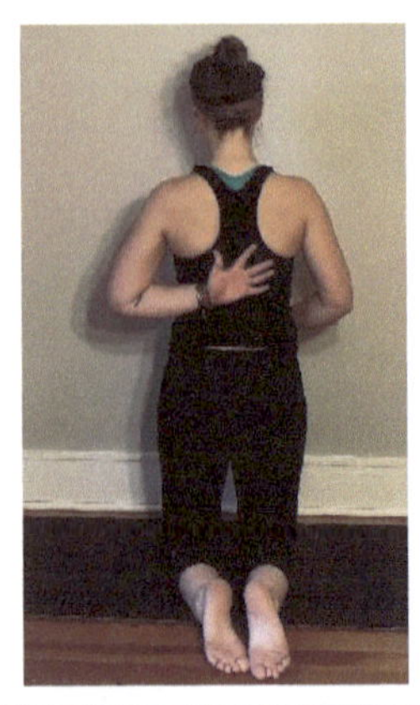

*Please note that Cable Rows and the Lat Pull Down exercises were done with a band but can be completed with a cable cord machine and/or the Lat pull down machine at your local gym. 2-3 sets of 10-15 for each to start. Play with lighter weights at first to help estabilsh the deep, foundational, stability muscles then work your way out!

27. Cable (Banded) Rows

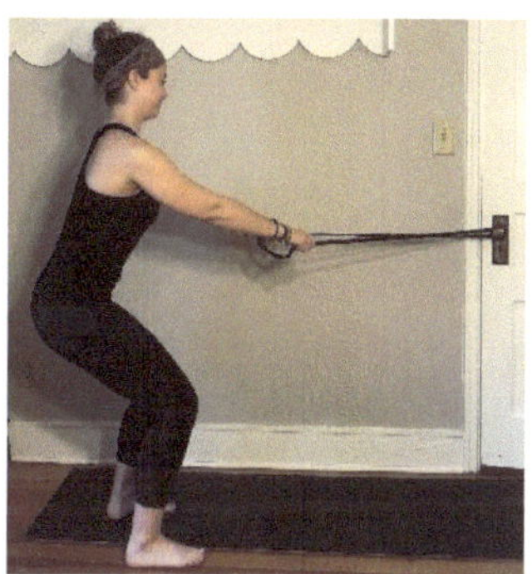
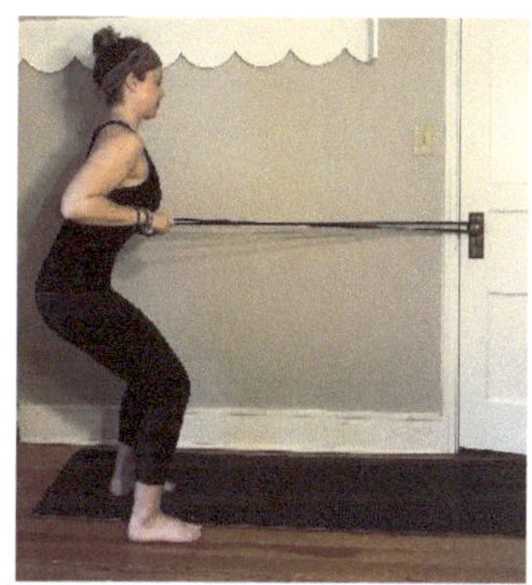

28. Bent over Row

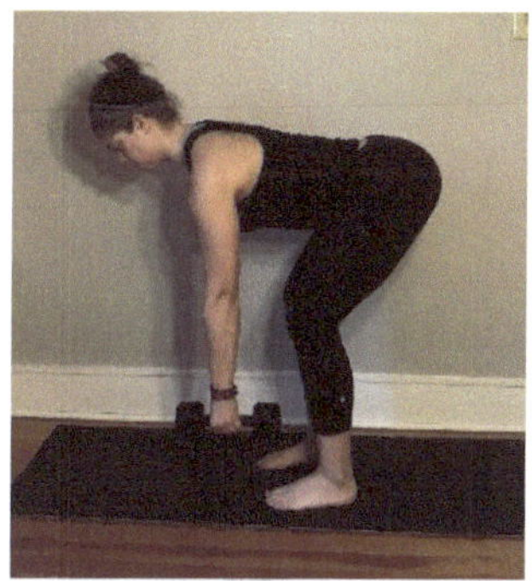
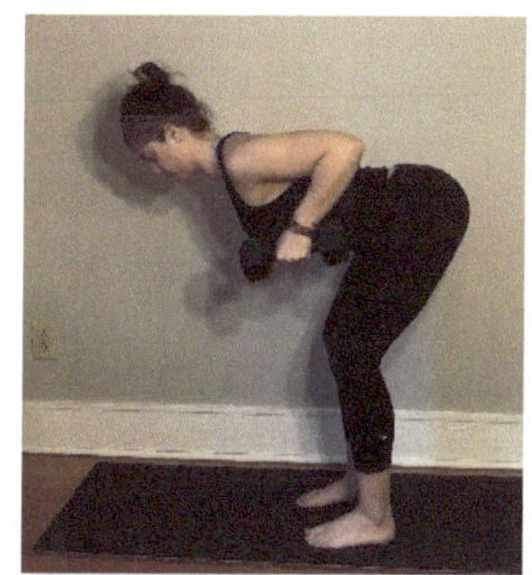

29. Lattisimus Dorsi "Lat" Pull Down

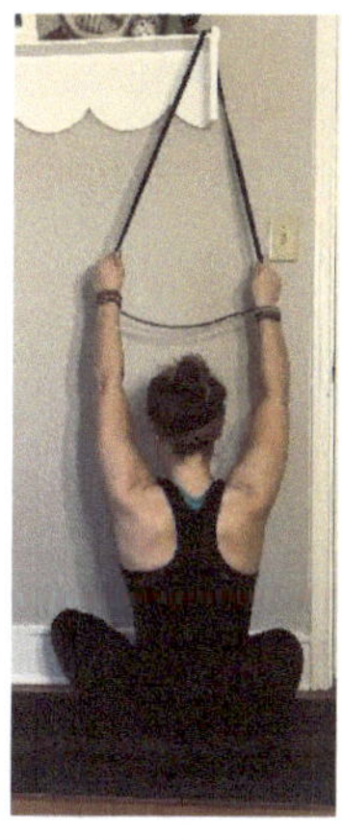
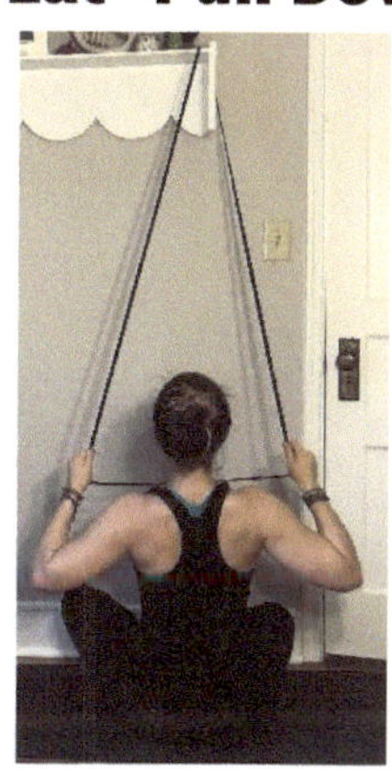

REFERENCES

Please note that this book was not pulled from one specific textbook, but rather a conglomeration of my knowledge throughout my education. Knowledge built through years of reading textbooks and evidence based research, conversations with other yogi's and medical professionals, ideas learned and worked through in workshops and teacher trainings that I've lead and attended.

With all that in mind, here is a list of some of my favorite Yoga Anatomy and Anatomy references:

Books:

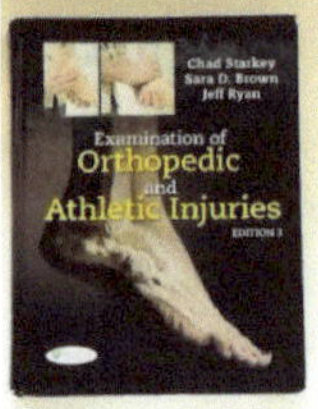

Examination of Orthopedic and Athletic Injuries by Chad Starkey, Sara Brown and Jeff Ryan – From my Athletic Training days. There is a TON of information in this book. Yoga instructors – this will be a lot of injury information you probably don't need to know. However, this book highlights the beginning of my career. It has muscle actions, innervations, origin and insertions in these neat little tables and special tests as well!

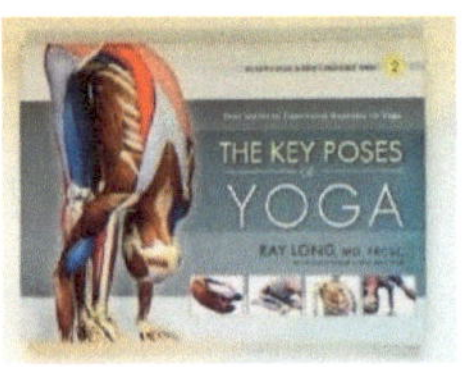
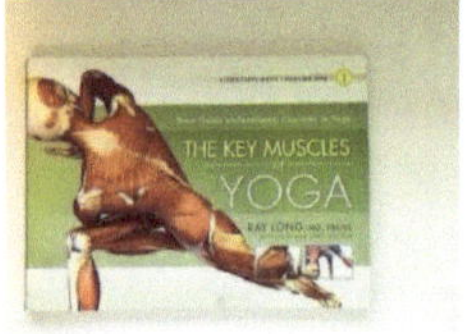

The Key Poses and the Key Muscles of Yoga books by Ray Long. He has a few more versions out there (backbends, hips, etc.) but these two are my favorites to use when I teach yoga anatomy weekends for teacher trainings. One of the most approachable anatomy books I've seen in a while! They hit on all the important parts! Plus, the graphics are on point!

Podcast:

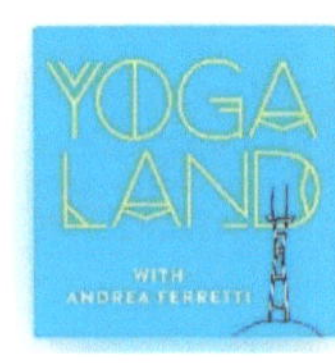

YogaLand by Andrea Ferretti

*The episodes with Jason Crandell always steal my anatomy heart!

www.ingramcontent.com/pod-product-compliance
Lightning Source LLC
Chambersburg PA
CBHW040043240726
48664CB00003B/1050